The 10-Day Paleo Challenge

by Anne Angelone

ISBN-13: 978-1484011805

ISBN-10: 1484011805

Disclaimer

This program manual is not intended to provide medical advice nor should it take the place of any medical advice or treatment from your personal physician.

Readers are advised to consult their own doctors or other qualified health professionals regarding the treatment of medical conditions.

The author shall not be held liable or responsible for any misunderstanding or misuse of the information contained in this program manual or for any loss, damage, or injury caused or alleged to be caused directly or indirectly by any treatment, action, or application of any food or food source discussed in this program manual.

The statements in this program manual have not been evaluated by the U.S. Food and Drug Administration.

This information is not intended to diagnose, treat, cure, or prevent any disease.

To request permission for reproduction or to inquire about private or group nutritional consulting or classes, please contact:

Anne Angelone, MS, Licensed Acupuncturist

website: www.anneangelone.com

Table of Content

Why go Paleo?

Food is medicine! Nearly all of the patients that I see in my acupuncture practice have hidden food sensitivities, which cause poor energy and digestion, brain fog, headaches, blood sugar, weight and skin problems. For all of these patients, I encourage a 10-Day Paleo Challenge with its built in avoidance of the major food allergens and inclusion of healthy and organic food. These patients suddenly start feeling great within a few days of The 10 Day Paleo Challenge! Why?

Think of your food as information going from your fork to your cells. What if your food is genetically modified, processed, or is a major allergen? What if you lack the digestive capacity to break down specific proteins, processed foods, or grains? If you are feeling inflamed, overweight and toxic, you must ask yourself the question: what kind of information are your cells receiving?

Some clues as to how your digestion is affecting you are seen in your skin, joints, digestion, energy, athletic performance, blood sugar swings and weight gain.

Paleo is the term used to revere the diet of our pre-agricultural ancestors since it was free of all the grains, processed foods, and sugars that seem to be causing the chronic diseases we face today. Whenever anyone removes these inflammatory foods from their diet, they report the benefits of weight loss, more stable blood sugar, better digestion, clearer skin, decreased inflammation, better sleep and a stronger immune system. Not bad for a simple change in dietary choices!

The 10-Day Paleo Challenge reflects a whole foods Paleo nutrition approach that outlines which foods to include and which foods to eliminate. Using this plan as a template, you will easily eliminate many of the major food allergens, stabilize your blood sugar, and decrease inflammation.

All of these guidelines just happen to result in better digestion, elimination, improved mental focus, improved mood, increased energy, less congestion, fewer allergic symptoms, less joint pain, increased sense of relaxation, enhanced sleep, and better athletic performance.

The 10 Day Challenge

The 10-Day Paleo Challenge allows everyone to experience the wellness that comes from eating clean, healthy, nutrient dense, unprocessed food. Of course, you are encouraged to continue on for longer. Most people will adopt this template for the long term due to the powerful benefits they receive. The dietary emphasis on whole, organic, and nutrient dense foods contributes to optimal digestion and immune function. Anti-inflammatory and antioxidant rich fruit and veggies are also part of this dietary emphasis. Blood sugar will stabilize and adrenals will strengthen by making use of the minerals and amino acids that come from both protein and veggies. Probiotic and cultured foods will help to reduce intestinal inflammation and provide the nutrients necessary for healthy intestinal micro-flora. Be sure to include lots of water and herbal teas, and you'll be off to a great start.

The most potent food required for the 10 Days can be found at the organic farmers market and the organic section of your health food store.

Emphasis is placed on blood sugar stabilization, hydration, and relaxation. 30 minutes of walking or exercising is imperative, and it will help you sleep 7-9 hours. After 10 Days, you will likely be feeling so recharged that you may want to continue. So, let's get started!

The 10 Day Paleo Challenge: Goals

Do's:

1. Eat organic pastured, grass fed animal protein, and wild fish.
2. Eat carbohydrates from fruits and vegetables.
3. Eat moderate fats from avocados, coconut, and olives.
4. Eat low glycemic fruits and non-starchy vegetables.
5. Eat fermented foods like sauerkraut, coconut kefir, and yogurt.
6. Stay hydrated with 8 glasses of water per day
7. Eat anti-inflammatory herbs and spices like turmeric and ginger.
8. Eat fiber from non-starchy fruits and vegetables.
9. Eat colorful veggies rich in plant phytonutrients, vitamins, minerals, and antioxidants.
10. Drink veggie, fish, chicken or beef bone broth daily.
11. Exercise every day, preferably for 30 minutes.
12. Practice awareness mindful of your breath for at least 5 minutes per day.
13. Take daily detox baths with Epsom salts and baking soda.
14. Drink green smoothies daily.
15. Consider digestive enzymes, hydrochloric acid, and apple cider vinegar to aid digestion.

Don'ts:

1. No grains at all.
2. No dairy products.
3. No genetically modified organism (GMO) foods.
4. No processed foods.
5. No sugars or dried fruits.
6. No cereals or grain like seeds.
7. No legumes (e.g. peanuts, beans, lentils, peas, and soybeans).
8. No nuts or seeds.
9. No fruit juices.
10. No skipping meals.

Benefits Of The 10 Day Paleo Challenge

HEALTHY FOODS

The 10-Day Paleo Challenge includes grass-fed, organic meats, wild fish, plenty of vegetables, healthy fats such as coconut oil, avocado, olive oil and salmon. The challenge also includes fermented foods such as sauerkraut, kefir, and coconut yogurt along with plenty of water and non-caffeinated herbal teas.

FINDING FOOD INTOLERANCES

Many people don't realize they have intolerance to food. Many foods trigger low energy, rashes, joint pain, digestive issues, headaches, anxiety, and even depression. The foods people most commonly react to are gluten, dairy, soy, corn, and sugary foods. You will be completely off these foods during the 10-Day Paleo Challenge; however, you may reintroduce them back into your diet in order to check your level of sensitivity after 10 days.

REWARDS

Better digestion and elimination, fewer symptoms of chronic illness, improved concentration, mental focus and clarity, improved mood, increased energy, less congestion, fewer allergic symptoms, less joint pain, increased sense of relaxation, and enhanced sleep.

WEIGHT LOSS

Many find that Paleo foods are great for weight loss. Cutting out sweets and high-carb foods naturally promote weight loss. Even more exciting, the Paleo food plan becomes a weight loss plan by reducing inflammation, stabilizing blood sugar, and restoring our adrenals glands.

The 10 Day Paleo Challenge

	Foods To Include	Foods To Eliminate
FRUITS	In Season, Organic, Fresh, and if possible, local; apple, apricot, banana, blackberry, boysenberry, cantaloupe, carambola, cassava melon cherimoya, cherries, cranberry, Figs, gooseberry, grapefruit, grapes, guava, honeydew, kiwi, lemon, lime, lychee, mango, nectarine, orange, papaya, passion fruit, peaches, pears, persimmons, pineapple, plums, pomegranate, raspberry, rhubarb, star fruit, strawberry, tangerine, watermelon.	**Avoid:** Dried and canned fruits.
VEGETABLES	All fresh raw, steamed, sautéed, juiced, or roasted vegetables. Asparagus, avocado, basil. beet, broccoli, cabbage, carrots, cauliflower, celery, chard, collards, cucumber, green beans, green onion, kale, kohlrabi, kumquats, lemons, lettuce, mushroom, mustard, okra, onions, spinach, summer squash, turnips, Artichoke hearts, Brussels sprouts, carrots, daikon, zucchini, fennel root, dandelion greens, bell pepper, cabbage.	**Avoid:** cassava root, manioc, tapioca, all potatoes except sweet potatoes

LEGUME	Legumes can irritate the gut lining, and are not part of the Paleo Challenge.	**Avoid:** All beans, black-eyed peas, cashews, chickpeas, lentils, miso, peas, peanuts/ peanut butter, soybean and soy products.
BREAD	Almond flour, coconut flour	**Avoid:** Corn, plus all gluten-containing grains and products including wheat, spelt, kamut, barley, rye, oat.
DENSE CARBS	Beets, acorn squash, butternut squash, yams, sweet potato.	**Avoid:** Cassava root, manioc, tapioca, all potatoes.

NUTS AND SEEDS	Almonds, cashews, walnuts, pumpkin seeds, brazil nuts, sunflower seeds, etc.,	**Avoid:** Peanuts, peanut butter.
MEAT	Beef, chicken; quail, squab, duck, goose, turkey, Cornish game hen; pasture-raised lamb, pork, buffalo/bison, goat, emu, ostrich, sausage (without fillers or nightshade spices); liver, kidney, heart, organic sliced meats (gluten, sugar free), uncured nitrate/nitrite-free deli meats and bacon from grass-fed/pastured beef/pork.	**Avoid:** Processed and canned meats: bacon, fatty cuts of lamb, beef, pork, deli meats, smoked/dried /salted meat and fish
WILD FISH	Salmon, mackerel, herring, halibut, shellfish, oysters, cod, tuna, flounder, sardines, hake, skate, trout, red snapper, etc.	**Avoid:** Whale, shark, swordfish. Farmed tilapia and catfish quantities should be moderate.

MILK AND YOGURT	Coconut milk, homemade almond, or other nut milk and yogurts.	**Avoid:** Cow and other animal (goat/sheep) milks, cheese, cottage cheese, cream, butter, yogurt, ice-cream, non-dairy creamers, soy milk, whey, butter, cheeses, frozen desserts, mayonnaise.
EGGS AND FATS	Omega 3 eggs. Good fats: olive oil, coconut oil, flaxseed, sesame, walnut, hazelnut oil, Coconut oil, lard, bacon grease, butter, ghee, tallow, duck fat, lamb fat.	**Avoid:** Margarine, butter, shortening, peanut oil, mayonnaise, any processed hydrogenated oils.
DRINKS	Filtered or distilled water, herbal tea, coffee, mineral water, broths, freshly made veggie juice, green smoothies, kefir water, coconut kefir, kombucha.	**Avoid:** Sodas and soft drinks, fruit juice.

SPICES	Ginger, rosemary, basil, cilantro, dill, ginger, lemongrass, peppermint, oregano, parsley, sage, sea, salt, thyme, tarragon, turmeric, spearmint, marjoram, mace, chives, chamomile, chervil, cinnamon, bay leaves, cloves, dill, horseradish, saffron, sea salt.	
CONDIMENTS	Apple cider vinegar, Balsamic vinegar, coconut vinegar, Red Boat fish sauce and coconut aminos, wasabi, mustard, horseradish, pesto.	**Avoid:** Ketchup, relish, soy sauce, BBQ sauce, chutneys, baker's yeast, brewer's yeast.
FERMENTED FOODS	Sauerkraut, pickled ginger, pickled cucumbers, coconut yogurt, coconut kefir, kefir water, kombucha, kimchi, pickles fermented with salt, beet kvass, lacto-fermented vegetables and fruits such as fermented beets, carrots, and green papaya.	
SUGARS	Honey, maple syrup, molasses, unrefined cane sugar, and date sugar.	**Avoid:** White or brown sugar, high fructose corn syrup, dried fruit. all sweeteners, including:

		Truvia, maple syrup, honey, agave, brown rice syrup, Splenda, Equal, Nutrasweet, xylitol, stevia.
ALL PROCESSED FOOD		**Avoid:** Cured meats, sugar, and sauces, mayonnaise, mustard, canned foods.

*Avoid any known food triggers, even if they are on the "Include" list.

The 10 Days

GETTING STARTED: THE BASICS

1. Include nutrient-dense foods such as grass fed organic protein sources, vegetables, and fats in your 3 daily meals.
2. Drink 8 glasses of water per day and include daily veggie broth.
3. Exercise every day, preferably for 30 minutes.
4. Relax with an awareness of your breathing for at least 5 minutes per day.
5. Take daily Detox baths with Epsom salts, baking soda, and lavender oil.
6. Drink green smoothies daily.

DAY 1:
Enjoy all "Foods to Include" and Recipes.
Hydrate with water, broths, and green smoothies. Exercise: for 30 minutes.

Enjoy: Detox baths, broths, meditation, and relaxation.

DAY 2:
Enjoy all "Foods to Include" and Recipes.
Hydrate with water, broths, and green smoothies.

Exercise: for 30 minutes.

Enjoy: Detox baths, broths, meditation, and relaxation.

DAY 3:
Enjoy all "Foods to Include" and Recipes.
Hydrate with water, broths, and green smoothies.

*Exercise:*for 30 minutes.

Enjoy: Detox baths, broths, meditation, and relaxation.

DAY'S 4 -10:

Keep going; you're doing great!

Enjoy all "Foods to Include" and Recipes. Hydrate with water, broths, and green smoothies

Exercise: for 30 minutes.

Enjoy: Detox Baths, Broths, Meditation, and Relaxation.

DAY 10:

Congratulations! You have successfully completed The 10-Day Paleo Challenge!

By continuing this diet and lifestyle, you'll maximize your benefits; these benefits include correcting your blood sugar problems, continuing to lose weight naturally, and reversing many other chronic problems.

Reintroducing Foods: Should you start reintroducing other foods and suspect that you may have food sensitivities, try just one new food at a time, and wait *72 hours* to see if you notice a reaction. If you're unsure about a reaction, wait until the symptoms recede, and eat only those foods that do not cause a reaction. You can then ingest the suspicious food again and take note.

The 10-Days for Grain Lovers

TRANSITIONING TO PALEO

If you need to make a gradual transition to the Paleo Diet, follow these suggestions to slowly wean yourself from sugar, grains, and processed foods.

The Basics:

1. Include nutrient-dense foods such as grass fed organic protein sources, vegetables, and fats in your 3 daily meals.
2. Drink 8 glasses of water per day and include daily veggie broth.
3. Exercise every day preferably for 30 minutes.
4. Relax with an awareness of your breathing for at least 5 minutes per day.
5. Take daily Detox baths with Epsom salts, baking soda, and lavender oil.
6. Drink green smoothies daily.

DAY 1:

Eliminate all: refined sugars & carbohydrates. This includes anything with added sucrose, high fructose corn syrup, alcohol, cakes, cookies, candies, pastries, beer, wine, liquor, or ice cream. This also includes any artificial colorings, flavorings, sweeteners, packaged, preserved, or processed foods.

Enjoy all "Foods to Include" and Recipes. Hydrate with water, broths and green smoothies.

Exercise: for 30 minutes.

Enjoy: Detox baths, broths, meditation, and relaxation.

DAY 2:

In addition to eliminating the foods listed for Day 1, eliminate all dairy products.

Enjoy all "Foods to Include" and Recipes. Hydrate with water, broths, and green, smoothies.

Exercise: for 30 minutes.

Enjoy: Detox baths, broths, meditation, and relaxation.

DAY 3:

In addition to eliminating foods listed for Days 1 & 2, eliminate: all gluten grains–wheat, oat, rye, barley, spelt, kamut, and bulgar, as well as corn & corn-derived foods.

Enjoy all "Foods to Include" and Recipes. Hydrate with water, broths and green smoothies.

Exercise: for 30 minutes.

Enjoy: Detox baths, broths, meditation, and relaxation.

DAY 4:

You are now in full-fledged Paleo mode.

Enjoy all "Foods to Include" and Recipes. Hydrate with water, broths and green smoothies.

Exercise: for 30 minutes.

Enjoy: Detox baths, broths, meditation and relaxation.

DAY'S 5-10:

Keep going; you're doing great!

Enjoy all "Foods to Include" and Recipes. Hydrate with water, broths and green smoothies.

Exercise: for 30 minutes.

Enjoy: Detox baths, broths, meditation and relaxation.

DAY 10:

Congratulations! You have successfully completed The 10-Day Paleo Challenge!

Consider using this Paleo template for 30 Days or longer! By continuing this diet and lifestyle, you'll maximize your benefits; these benefits include correcting your blood sugar problems, continuing to lose weight naturally and reversing many other chronic problems.

Reintroducing Foods: Should you start reintroducing foods and suspect that you may have food sensitivities, try just one new food at a time, and wait 72 hours to see if you notice a reaction. If you're unsure about a reaction, wait until the symptoms recede, and eat only those foods that do not cause a reaction. You can then ingest the suspicious food again and take note.

The 10 Day Paleo Challenge Menu!

The 10 Day Paleo Challenge Menu					
	Breakfast	**Snack**	**Lunch**	**Snack**	**Dinner**	**Beverage**
Day 1	Stir Fried Chicken Bread with zucchini and basil	Green Smoothie	Arugula Salas with Grilled Trip-Tip	GreenSalad with jicama, cucumber and steamed carrots	Ginger Steamed Halibut with sautéed mustad greens	Kombucha
Day 2	Ground beef sautéed in olive oil with salt, oregano, diced carrots and kale	Chicken Liver Pate with carrot sticks	Seared Mackerel with wasabi and side of mustard greens	Bone Broth with spinach and basil	Slow Cooked Chicken	Water
Day 3	Turkey sausage with steamed Bok Choy	Sliced turkey breast with slices of cucumber	Jumbo Shrimp sautééed with watercress	Veggie Broth	Turmeric Chicken with sautéed zucchini, cucumber/dill salad	Rooilboos Tea
Day 4	Turkey patties with sauteed Rainbow chard	Blueberry Coconut kedir water	Grilled Chicken wrapped in steamed collard with crunchy veggies	Bone Broth	Rosemary and Sea Salt Baked Lamb Chops and arugula salad	Water with 1 Tbsp Apple Cider Vinegar
Day 5	Home Made Coconut Yogurt with bananaand blueberries	Fermented carrots with cucumbers, chicken breast slices	Grill Pan Pork Chops sautedd yellow squash, kixed green salad.	Grapefruit	Balsamic Pork Tendeloin	Mint Tea
Day 6	Pork sausages sautéed with Swiss chard	Veggie Broth	Crock Pot Chicken	Home Made coconut yogurt	Wasabi Tuna Steak sauteed spinach and romaine salad	Green Smoothie
Day 7	Roast beef slices, Green Smoothie	Bacon, spinach salad with grated carrot, balsamic, olive oil, sea salt	Bacon, Arugula, Daikon and Carrot Salad	Chicken breast slices	Grilled Rosemary Dijon Salmon Steak with steamed Lacninato kale	Kombucha
Day 8	Grilled Rosemary Dijon Salmon Steak with steamed Lacinato kale	Orange slices, 2 .oz grilled chicken breast.	Seared Mackerel with mustard greens	GreenSalad with jicama, cucumber and steamed carrots	Bacon Wrapped Chicken Thighs with steamed Buttermut squash	Kombucha
Day 9	Chicken sausage sauteed with water chestnuts and Swiss chard	Cucumber with sea salt, turkey breast	Pan Seared Yellowtail with sautéed spinach	Bone Broth	Balsamic Marinated Pork Chop with mashed turnips and sautéed greens	Water with Lemon
Day 10	Chicken breast sautéed with coconut aminos, Bok Choy	Lemon Urange Gelatino	Raw zucchini noodles with seasoned ground pork	Veggie Broth	Tueric Chicken with zucchini and butter leaf salad	Ginger Tea

Day 1

- STIR FRIED CHICKEN BREAST WITH ZUCCHINI AND BASIL
- GREEN SMOOTHIE
- ARUGULA SALAD WITH GRILLED TRI-TIP
- GREEN SALAD WITH JICAMA, CUCUMBER AND STEAMED CARROTS
- GINGER STEAMED HALIBUT WITH SAUTÉED MUSTARD GREENS

Day 2

- CHICKEN LIVER PATE WITH CARROT STICKS
- SEARED MACKEREL WITH WASABI AND SIDE OF MUSTARD GREENS
- BONE BROTH WITH SPINACH AND BASILSLOW COOKED CHICKEN

Day 3

- JUMBO SHRIMP SAUTÉED WITH WATERCRESS
- VEGGIE BROTH
- Turmeric Chicken with zucchini and basil

Day 4

- BLUEBERRY COCONUT KEFIR WATER
- GRILLED CHICKEN WRAPPED IN STEAMED COLLARD WITH CRUNCHY VEGGIES
- BONE BROTH
- ROSEMARY AND SEA SALT BAKED LAMB CHOPS; AND ARUGULA SALAD

Day 5

- Homemade Coconut yogurt
- Balsamic pork tenderloin on a bed of Red Kale
- Grill pan pork chops with sauteed Yellow Squash and Arugula Salad

Day 6

- Vegetable broth
- Homemade Coconut yogurt
- Green Smoothie with Blueberry, kale, ginger

Day 7

- Green Smoothie with Blueberry, kale, ginger
- Bacon Arugula Daikon and carrot salad
- Grilled Rosmary Salmon steak with steamed Lacinato Kale

Day 8

- Grilled Rosmary Salmon steak with steamed Lacinato Kale
- Seared mackerel with wasabi and side of mustard greens
- GREEN SALAD WITH JICAMA, CUCUMBER AND STEAMED CARROTS
- Bacon Wrapped Chicken Thighs

Day 9

- Pan Seared yellowtail with sauteed spinach
- Bone broth
- Balsamic marinated pork chops with mashed turnips and sauteed collards

Day 10

- Lemon Orange Gelatino
- Raw zucchini noodles with seasoned ground pork
- Vegetable broth
- Stir fried chicken WITH yellow summer squash and mint
- Turmeric Chicken with zucchini and basil

MENU

FISH

- Pan Seared yellowtail with sauteed spinach

BEEF

- Pastured Tri-Tip, Jumbo Shrimp and collard greens

POULTRY

- Bacon Wrapped Chicken Thighs
- Stir fried chicken WITH yellow summer squash and mint
- Turmeric Chicken with zucchini and basil
- Chicken Liver Pate
- Slow cooked chicken
- Grilled chicken wrapped in steamed collard greens with crunchy Veggies

SOUP

- Vegetable broth
- Bone broth

PORK

- Balsamic marinated pork chops with mashed turnips and sauteed collards
- Grill pan pork chops with sauteed Yellow Squash and Arugula Salad
- Balsamic pork tenderloin on a bed of Red Kale
- Balsamic marinated pork chops with mashed turnips and sauteed collards
- Raw zucchini noodles with seasoned ground pork

SALADS

- Bacon Arugula Daikon and carrot salad
- NEw York Steak and Spinach Salad
- Cucumber, Nori salad
- Grilled Tri-Tip with Arugula Salad

EAFOOD

- Seared mackerel with wasabi and side of mustard greens
- Grilled Rosmary Salmon steak with steamed Lacinato Kale
- Jumbo Shrimp Sauteed with watercress
- Steamed Alaskan King crab with sauteed bok choy
- Ginger Steamed Halibut and sauteed Mustard greens
- Seared mackerel with wasabi and side of mustard greens

DRINKS

- Green Smoothie with Blueberry, kale, ginger
- Blueberry coconut Kefir water

LAMB

- Rosemary and Sea Salt baked Lamb Chops on a bed of Kale Chips

DESSERTS

- Homemade Coconut yogurt
- Lemon Orange Gelatino

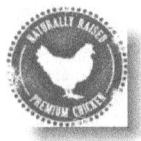

BACON WRAPPED CHICKEN THIGHS

- 4 pieces of boneless, skinless chicken thighs
- 4 pieces of bacon
- 3 Tbsp olive oil
- 1 tsp sea salt

Preparation

1. Preheat the oven to 375 F.
2. Coat chicken with olive oil and salt, fold in half then wrap one piece of bacon around each chicken thigh.
3. Bake for 30 minutes. Broil the chicken for another 5-10 minutes or until the bacon is crispy and the chicken is fully cooked.
4. Servings: 2

TURMERIC CHICKEN WITH ZUCCHINI AND BASIL

- 2 grilled chicken breasts
- 3 medium zucchinis, sliced thinly
- ½ bunch of basil leaves
- 2 Tbsp olive oil
- 2 tsp Turmeric
- Olive oil spray
- Sea salt to taste

Preparation

1. Coat chicken breasts with olive oil spray and salt and turmeric. Grill for 8-10 minutes on each side.
2. Sautee zucchini in olive oil for 10 minutes and add basil in last 2 minutes.
3. Slice chicken and serve with sautéed zucchini.
4. Servings: 2

STIR FRIED CHICKEN BREAST
WITH YELLOW SUMMER SQUASH AND MINT IN BUTTER LEAF LETTUCE WRAP

1. 2 chicken breasts
2. 3 medium zucchinis, sliced thinly
3. 1/2 bunch of mint
4. 4 Tbsp olive oil
5. Olive oil spray
6. Sea salt to taste
7. 1 head of butter leaf lettuce

Preparation

1. Cut chicken into cubes and sauté in olive oil, pinch of salt.
2. After 5 minutes add zucchini in olive oil and sauté for 7 minutes
3. Fill butter leaf lettuce with sauté and fresh mint, serve.
4. Servings: 2-3

CHICKEN LIVER PATE

- 1 pound chicken livers
- 1/3 cup olive oil
- 2 tbsp capers
- 2 Tbsp Dijon mustard
- 3 tsp fresh thyme
- 2 tsp fresh rosemary
- ¼ cup beef broth or water
- Sea salt to taste

Preparation

1. Sauté chicken livers in olive oil until brown.
2. Add broth, herbs, capers and Dijon mustard and simmer until liquid is mostly gone.
3. Add salt to taste, blend in Cuisinart, refrigerate.

SLOW COOKED CHICKEN

- 3 Lbs boneless, skinless chicken thighs
- 3 parsnips, chopped
- 3 carrots, chopped
- 4 celery stalks
- Sea salt to taste
- 2 medium zucchinis chopped
- 1/4 cup olive oil
- 1 TB dried thyme
- 1 TB sage
- 1 1/2 cups chicken broth

Preparation

1. Add everything to your slow cooker or crock-pot and let cook on medium-high for 4 hours.

GRILLED CHICKEN WRAPPED IN STEAMED COLLARD GREENS
WITH CRUNCHY VEGGIES

- 2 chicken breasts
- 1 Tbsp coconut aminos
- 1 Tbsp minced ginger
- 3 large carrots, peeled and diced
- Sea salt
- 2 Tbsp olive oil
- ½ daikon radish, peeled and diced
- 2 ribs of celery, chopped
- 1 bunch of collard greens

Preparation

1. Marinate chicken breast in olive oil, coconut aminos and ginger for 1 hour or longer.
2. Cut veggies, steam collard greens
3. Grill chicken breasts for 12 minutes each side making sure thoroughly cooked.

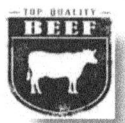

PASTURED TRI-TIP, JUMBO SHRIMP AND COLLARD GREENS

- 1 pound Tri-Tip steak
- ½ pound pre-cooked shrimp
- 1 bunch of collard greens, rolled then cut thin
- 5 Tbsp olive oil
- Sea salt to taste

Preparation

1. 1 Lightly salt Tri-tip and grill for 7 minutes on each side.
2. 2 Sautee collard greens in olive oil add shrimp for 5 minutes
3. 3 Sprinkle salt on Tri-tip and cook on grill pan
4. Servings: 1-2

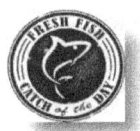

PAN SEARED YELLOWTAIL WITH SAUTEED SPINACH

- 1 pound yellow tail
- 2 Tbsp olive or red palm oil
- 1 bunch of spinach
- 2 Tbsp coconut aminos
- 1 Tbsp minced ginger
- Sea salt to taste

Preparation

1. Marinate yellowtail ginger, coconut aminos and olive oil for 1 hour.
2. Sautee spinach in olive oil with salt to taste.
3. Spray and preheat skillet on med-high for 3 minutes.
4. Add yellow tail and cook for one minute per ½ inch of thickness,

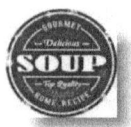

VEGETABLE BROTH

- 3 quarts of water
- 2 sliced carrots
- 1 cup of cubed daikon
- 1 cup of turnips and rutabaga cut into large cubes
- 2 cups of chopped greens: kale, parsley, collard greens, chard, dandelion, cilantro
- 2 celery stalks
- 4 ½ inch slices of ginger

Preparation

1. Add all the ingredients at once and place on low boil for 60 minutes.
2. Cool and strain veggies out-discard them.
3. Store in fridge. Heat and drink 3-4 cups/day.
4. Servings: 8 cups

BONE BROTH

- 4 quarts water
- 2 lbs chicken or beef bones (or oxtail)
- 3 ribs of celery
- 2 bay leaves
- 2 tablespoon apple cider vinegar
- 1 teaspoon sea salt

Preparation

1. Place all ingredients in pot and bring the stock to a boil, then reduce the heat to low and allow the stock to cook from 8 hours.
2. Allow the stock to cool then strain to discard bones etc.
3. Store your stock in the fridge and use within a few days.
4. Servings: 1-2

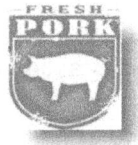

BALSAMIC MARINATED PORK CHOPS
WITH MASHED TURNIPS AND SAUTEED COLLARDS

- 1 teaspoon sea salt
- 1/4 cup balsamic vinegar
- 6 Tbsp olive oil divided
- 2 bone in one pork chops
- 1 bunch of collard greens
- 4 turnip, boiled until soft
- Sea salt to taste

Preparation

1. Marinate chops for at least one and up to 24 hours in balsamic vinegar and 2 Tbsp Olive oil.
2. Grill 7 minutes per side, checking for doneness
3. While turnips are boiling, sauté the collard greens in olive oil.
4. Mash turnip, add a dash of olive oil and salt to taste

RAW ZUCCHINI NOODLES WITH SEASONED GROUND PORK

- 2 large zucchinis, julienned
- ½ pound ground pork
- ¼ bunch chopped fresh basil
- ¼ bunch chopped fresh oregano
- Sea salt to taste
- Tbsp olive oil

Preparation

1. Sautee basil, oregano and pork in olive oil until fully cooked, add salt to taste.
2. Pour on top of zucchini pasta; add more fresh basil, Enjoy!

GRILL PAN PORK CHOPS
WITH SAUTEED YELLOW SQUASH AND ARUGULA SALAD

- 2 Pork Chops
- 5 small yellow squash sliced
- ¼ bunch of fresh flat leaf parsley
- 5 Tbsp olive oil divided
- 2 Tbsp balsamic vinegar
- 4 cups arugula
- Sea salt to taste

Preparation

1. Mix thyme with olive oil and salt to rub chops.
2. Grill on med-high heat for 5-7 minutes per side.
3. Sautee yellow squash in olive oil with parsley.
4. Mix arugula with 2 Tbsp Olive oil and 2 Tbsp balsamic vinegar.
5. Servings: 2

BALSAMIC PORK TENDERLOIN ON A BED OF RED KALE

- 1 teaspoon salt
- 1/4 cup balsamic vinegar
- 1/2 cup olive oil
- 1 one pound pork tenderloin
- 6 leaves of Russian red kale

Preparation

1. Marinate pork for at least one hour and up to 24 hours in above ingredients.
2. Spray olive oil in a baking dish.
3. Massage kale leaves with olive oil and a sprinkle of salt.
4. Pan sears the tenderloin then place on top of kale.
5. Bake in oven at 350F for 25 minutes or to desired doneness.
6. Be sure to eat the kale chips!

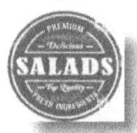

GREEN SMOOTHIE
WITH BLUEBERRY, KALE, GINGER

- 1/2 a bunch Dino kale or Swiss chard, cut out stalks
- 1/2 inch ginger
- ½ cup blueberries
- 5 cups of water
- Blend for 5 minutes

BACON ARUGULA DAIKON AND CARROT SALAD

- 2 strips of bacon, cooked and chopped
- 1 head of arugula
- 1 small daikon radish, grated
- 1 carrot, grated
- 2 Tbsp olive oil
- 1 tsp sea salt
- 1 Tbsp apple cider vinegar

Preparation

1. Mix arugula with grated daikon, carrots in a large bowl.
2. Stir in the olive oil, vinegar, salt, adjust seasonings.
3. Servings: 1-2

NEW YORK STEAK AND SPINACH SALAD

- 1 pound New York Steak
- 1 head of washed spinach
- ½ cup grated jicama plus 1 carrot peeled and grated
- ½ peeled and sliced cucumber
- 2 Tbsp olive oil
- 2 Tbsp balsamic vinegar
- Sea salt to taste
- olive oil spray

Preparation

1. Mix spinach with grated jicama, carrots in a large bowl.
2. Stir in olive oil, vinegar, and salt.
3. Sprinkle sea salt and spray olive oil on New York Steak, cook on grill pan for 7 minutes per side. Slice and serve over salad.
4. Servings: 2

CUCUMBER, NORI SALAD

- 2 Nori sheets
- 1 cucumber, peeled, seeded and sliced thin
- 2 Tbsp apple cider vinegar
- 1 tsp ginger root, chopped
- Juice of ½ a lime
- I carrot sliced thin
- 1 tsp. coconut aminos
- 1 Tbsp olive oil
- Sea salt to taste

Preparation

1. Prepare carrot, ginger and cucumber.
2. Cut Nori into thin strips and let sit in a bowl of warm water.
3. Combine the coconut aminos, olive oil, sea salt and apple cider vinegar.
4. Pour over cut veggies, remove Nori from water and add to salad.
5. Servings: 1-2

GRILLED TRI-TIP WITH ARUGULA SALAD

- 4 cups fresh arugula
- ½ cup peeled and grated jicama
- 1 carrot peeled and grated
- 2 Tbsp olive oil
- 2 Tbsp balsamic vinegar
- Sea salt to taste
- ½ pound Tri-tip steak

Preparation

1. Mix arugula with grated, jicama carrots in a large bowl.
2. Stir in the olive oil, vinegar, salt, and Adjust seasonings.
3. Sprinkle salt on Tri-Tip steak and cook on grill pan for 7-10 minutes on each side.
4. Servings: 1-2

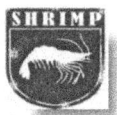

SEARED MACKEREL
WITH WASABI AND SIDE OF MUSTARD GREENS

- 2 Tbsp coconut aminos
- 1 pound mackerel
- 2 Tbsp ginger
- 4 cups mustard greens
- 2 Tbsp olive or red palm oil
- 2 tsp wasabi powder
- Olive oil spray
- 2 Tbsp fresh cilantro (chopped)
- Pinch of sea salt

Preparation

1. Marinate mackerel in coconut aminos, olive oil and wasabi powder.
2. Grill for 5 minutes on each side.
3. Sautee spinach in oil, sea salt to taste.
4. Servings: 1-2

GRILLED ROSMARY SALMON STEAK WITH STEAMED LACINATO KALE

- 1 bunch Lacinato aka Dino Kale
- 1 pound salmon
- 2 sprigs rosemary
- 2 Tbsp olive or red palm oil
- Olive oil spray
- Sea salt to taste

Preparation

1. Coat the salmon with olive oil spray, a light dusting of salt and crushed rosemary. Grill for 8 minutes on each side.
2. Steam kale and serve.
3. Servings: 2

JUMBO SHRIMP SAUTEED WITH WATERCRESS

- 1/2 cup chicken stock or broth
- 1/4 cup Red Boat fish sauce
- 5 tablespoons olive oil
- 1 1/4 pounds shelled and deveined jumbo shrimp
- 3 tablespoons minced fresh ginger
- One 6-ounce bunch watercress
- 1 tablespoon fresh lime juice

Preparation

1. In a small bowl, whisk together the stock, fish sauce.
2. In a large skillet, heat 2 tablespoons of olive oil. Add shrimp and cook over high heat, turning once, about 1 minute per side. Transfer to a plate.
3. Add the remaining 3 tablespoons of oil to the skillet. Add ginger and stir-fry over high heat until fragrant, about 1 minute.

4. Stir the stock mixture, add it to the skillet and bring to a boil. Stir in the watercress, then the shrimp and lime juice. Transfer the stir-fry to bowls.

GINGER STEAMED HALIBUT AND SAUTEED MUSTARD GREENS

- 1 pound halibut
- 1 inch of sliced ginger
- ¼ bunch cilantro
- Lemon slices
- 2 Tbsp olive or red palm oil
- 2 tbsp coconut aminos
- Sea salt to taste
- One bunch of mustard greens

Preparation

1. Cover Halibut with olive oil, coconut aminos, cilantro, lemon and ginger.
2. Steam the fish for 15 minutes.
3. Sauté mustard greens in olive oil, add salt to taste.
4. Servings: 2

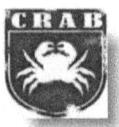

STEAMED ALASKAN KING CRAB
WITH SAUTEED BOK CHOY

- Alaskan king crab claws
- One bunch of Bok Choy
- ½ bunch of cilantro chopped
- 6 Tbsp red palm oil, divided
- Sea salt to taste

Preparation

1. Chop cilantro and mix or blend with 3 Tbsp olive oil.
2. Bring a large pot of water to a boil. Place thawed or fresh crab in a steamer for 10 minutes. Then crack them open and drizzle with olive oil, cilantro blend.
3. Sautee Bok Choy in olive oil, add salt to taste and serve with King Crab.
4. Servings: 1-2

BLUEBERRY COCONUT KEFIR WATER

- 1 quart coconut water
- 1 cup blueberries
- Tbsp dairy free water kefir grains

Preparation

1. Place water kefir grains in coconut water.
2. Cover jar loosely and set aside for at least 24hours.
3. Remove the Kefir Grains.
4. Puree blueberries with coconut kefir water in a blender.

HOMEMADE COCONUT YOGURT

- 1-quart coconut milk
- ¼ tsp probiotic yogurt starter
- Yogurt maker

Preparation

1. Heat a quart of unsweetened coconut milk to 105F - 110F.
2. Add ¼ teaspoon of yogurt starter and pulse 2x with the blender. You can add more than 1/4 teaspoon per quart if a very firm yogurt is desired.
3. Plug in your yogurt maker and pour the mixture into your yogurt maker container or containers and ferment for 12 hours.
4. Place in refrigerator for 4 hours.

LEMON ORANGE GELATINO

- Juice from 1 orange
- 1 tsp lemon zest
- 1 tsp grated orange zest
- 1 cup boiling water
- 4 Tbsp unflavored gelatin

Preparation

1. Mix orange juice, lemon and orange zest, set aside.
2. Add 1 cup boiling water to 4 tablespoons of gelatin in a bowl.
3. Strain lemon and orange zest from juice and add to gelatin.
4. Stir until well blended and then set aside to cool.
5. Pour into a glass dish or molds and refrigerate for 60 minutes.

SEARED MACKEREL
WITH WASABI AND SIDE OF MUSTARD GREENS

- 2 Tbsp coconut aminos
- 1 pound mackerel
- 2 Tbsp ginger
- 4 cups mustard greens
- 2 Tbsp olive or red palm oil
- 2 tsp wasabi powder
- Olive oil spray
- 2 Tbsp fresh cilantro (chopped)
- Pinch of sea salt

Preparation

1. Marinate mackerel in coconut aminos, olive oil and wasabi powder.
2. Grill for 5 minutes on each side.
3. Sautee spinach in oil, sea salt to taste.
4. Servings: 1-2

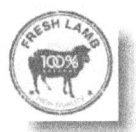

ROSEMARY AND SEA SALT BAKED LAMB CHOPS
ON A BED OF KALE CHIPS WITH ARUGULA AND ENDIVE SALAD

INGREDIENTS:

- 1 pound lamb chops
- 2 Tbsp minced fresh rosemary
- 2 teaspoons sea salt
- 4 Tbsp olive oil, divided
- 5 pieces of Kale
- Olive oil spray
- 1 head of arugula
- 6 heads of endive
- 1 cucumber, sliced
- 1 Tbsp. balsamic vinegar

Preparation

1. Rub chops with olive oil, rosemary and sea salt.
2. Spray olive oil in a baking dish.
3. Coat 5 large kale leaves with olive oil.
4. Place lamb chops on top of Kale
5. Bake in oven @ 375F for 20 minutes, turn chops over, and cook for 20 more minutes, or to desired doneness.
6. Toss arugula, endive and cucumber with olive oil and sea salt to taste.
7. Be sure to eat the kale chips!
8. Servings: 2-3

TRANSITIONING TO PALEO DETOX SUPPORT

DETOX BATH

- 2 cups of Epsom Salts plus
- 1 cup of baking soda
- 10 drops of lavender essential oil

DETOX BROTH

- 3 quarts of water
- 1 large chopped onion
- 2 sliced carrots
- 1 cup of daikon
- 1 cup of turnips and rutabaga cut into large cubes
- 2 cups of chopped greens: kale, parsley, beet greens, collard greens, chard, dandelion, cilantro or other greens
- 2 celery stalks
- 1/2 cup of cabbage
- 4 1/2 inch slices of ginger
- 2 cloves of whole garlic sea salt to taste

Preparation

1. Add all the ingredients at once and place on low boil for 60 minutes. Cool and strain the veggies out, then discard them.
2. Makes approximately 8 cups. Store in fridge. Heat and drink 3-4 cups/day.

LIVER DETOX

Olive oil & lemon juice (one tablespoon of each mixed with 4 oz. of water)

RAW APPLE CIDER VINEGAR

1 tablespoon diluted with 1 tablespoon water helps your stomach produce hydrochloric acid, and aid digestion of proteins.

EASY EXERCISE

30 minute walk per day

ADDITIONAL NUTRITIONAL SUPPLEMENTS

Consider depending on your needs

- Acidophilus
- Digestive enzymes
- Hydrochloric acid
- Omega 3 fatty acids
- Fiber

Conclusion

Here we are at the end the The 10-Day Paleo Challenge. If you are serious about your health and would like to join a group of amazing people on the same Paleo path, head over to my website and check out my <u>classes</u> page for the next set of group coaching tele-classes and to participate in a 30 Day Paleo Challenge.

Good Luck and have fun!

About The Author

Anne Angelone, Licensed Acupuncturist
Bachelor of Science, Cornell University
Master of Science, American College of Traditional Chinese Medicine
Member of Primal Docs
The Paleo Physician's Network
And Dr. Kharrazian's Thyroid Docs

✦ Background ✦

My own experience with Ankylosing Spondylitis (AS) led me to study the underlying mechanisms of disease expression. Since Ankylosing Spondylitis is correlated with the gene type called HLA B-27, I learned how to identify and remove specific triggers and then how to heal my leaky gut. I also learned how it's possible to turn off inflammatory gene expression with nutrition, supplements, Qi (oxygen), acupuncture, exercise, diet, and meditation. I am grateful to be able to share what I have learned through experience, years of research, training, and investigation.

My background in Functional Medicine has included advanced training with Dr. Datis Kharrazian in Functional Blood Chemistry Analysis, Mastering the Thyroid, Neurotransmitters and the Brain, Functional Endocrinology, Autoimmunity and Gluten Sensitivity. My hope is to share this information with those who would like to treat the underlying causes of "chronic symptoms" and experience greater health sooner, rather than later.

For more info contact: www.anneangelone.com

Other titles by Anne Angelone

The Autoimmune Paleo Plan
The Autoimmune Diet
The Paleo Autoimmune Protocol

Paleo Recommendations:

I highly recommend Chris Kresser's Personal Paleo Code (which has the option of a meal plan generator that you can customize) and Diane Sanfilippo's new book, Practical Paleo, which is one of my favorites. Check out the Paleo page on my Paleo website for links to these and more Paleo Nutrition guides.

Sarah Ballantyne, Ph.D. aka: The Paleo Mom
Practical Paleo by Diane Sanfilippo And Balanced Bites
Chris Kresser's: Personal Paleo Code

The Paleo Parents Pinterest page

Please check out Sarah Ballantyne's, book The Paleo Approach: Reverse Autoimmune Disease and Heal Your Body, available for pre-order on Amazon.

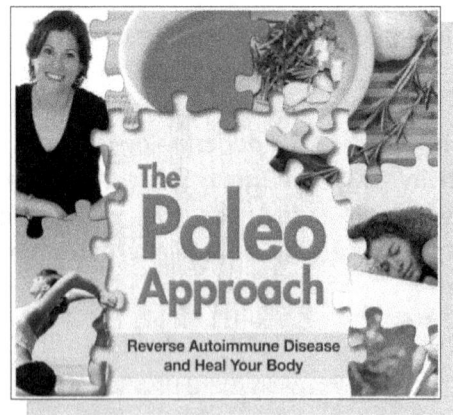

www.ingramcontent.com/pod-product-compliance
Lightning Source LLC
Chambersburg PA
CBHW070403290526
45790CB00004B/1620